NATURAL ANTI-INFLAMMATORY REMEDIES

CARMA books

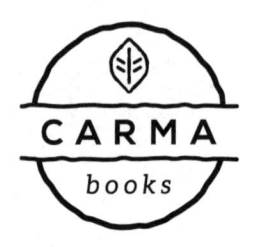

'A conscious approach to health & nutrition'

carmabooks.com

You are invited to to join our **Free Book Club** *mailing list. Sign up via our website to receive* **special offers** *and* **free for a limited time** *Health & Wellness eBooks!*

NATURAL ANTI-INFLAMMATORY REMEDIES

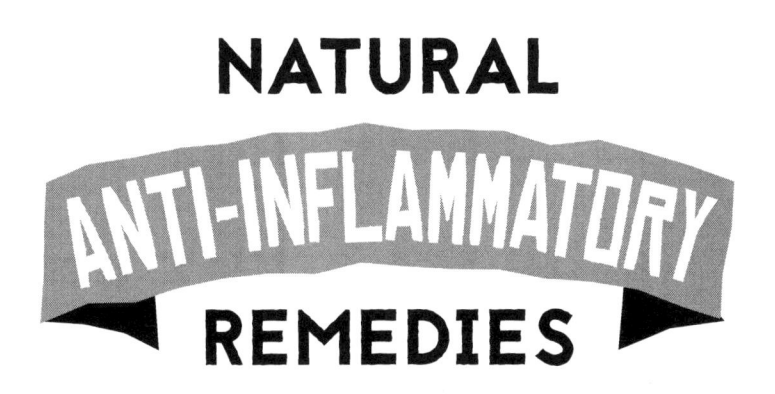

A COMPLETE GUIDE
to Inflammation + Healing with Holistic Herbs, Diet + Supplements

Carmen Reeves

Copyright © 2015 Carma Books

All rights reserved. No part of this publication may be reproduced, distributed, or transmitted in any form or by any means, including photocopying, recording, or other electronic or mechanical methods, without the prior written permission of the publisher.

Disclaimer

This book provides general information and extensive research regarding health and related subjects. The information provided in this book, and in any linked materials is for informational purposes only, and is not intended to be construed as medical advice. Speak with your physician or other healthcare professional before taking any nutritional or herbal supplements. There are no 'typical' results from the information provided - as individuals differ, the results will differ. Before considering any guidance from this book, please ensure you do not have any underlying health conditions which may interfere with the suggested healing methods. If the reader or any other person has a medical concern or pre-existing condition, he or she should consult with an appropriately licensed physician or healthcare professional. Never disregard professional medical advice or delay in seeking it because of something you have read in this book or in any linked materials.

Carma Books
carmabooks.com

hello@carmabooks.com

CONTENTS

INTRODUCTION 8

CHAPTER 1

What is Inflammation? 13

Symptoms of Inflammation 14
Types of Inflammation (Acute & Chronic) 16
The Immune System 19
Mast Cells 20
Histamines 21
C-Reactive Protein 22
The Liver 22

CHAPTER 2

What Causes Inflammation? 24

Infection and Injury 24
Burns 25
Common Illnesses 26
Allergens 27
Poor Diet and Bad Foods 27
Toxins and Alcohol 28
Overexertion/Overuse 29
Immune System Dysfunction 30
Stress 30

CHAPTER 3

Why is Minimizing Inflammation Vital to our Overall Health? 33

Inflammation and the Digestive System 33
Inflammation and the Heart/Blood Vessels 34
Inflammation and the Respiratory System 35
Inflammation and the Urinary System 36
Inflammation and the Skeletal System 36
Inflammation and the Muscular System 37
Inflammation and the Nervous System 38
Inflammation and the Immune System 39

CHAPTER 4

Conditions and Illnesses Related to Inflammation 41

The meaning of the suffix "-itis" 42
Minor Ailments Related to Inflammation 43
Major Illnesses Related to Inflammation 46

CHAPTER 5

How Can I Avoid and Heal Inflammation? 50

Foods to Avoid 51
Foods to Emphasize 54
Herbal Healing, Supplements and Lifestyle/Diet Tips for Inflammatory Conditions 58

THANK YOU 70
A WORD FROM THE PUBLISHER 72

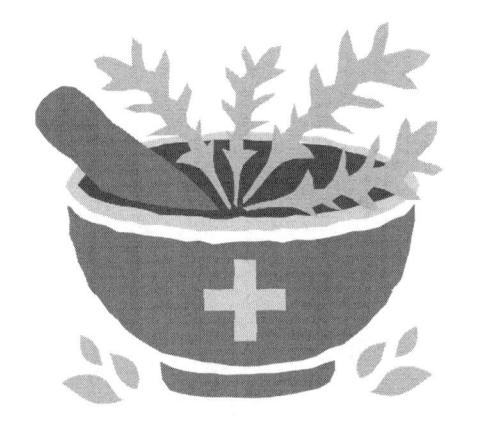

INTRODUCTION

Thank you and congratulations on your purchase of *Natural Anti-Inflammatory Remedies: A Complete Guide to Inflammation & Healing with Holistic Herbs, Diet & Supplements.* You've come to the right book if you are feeling like inflammation could have a large hand in your health struggles, just as I once did. **Let this be your guide and first step towards getting better health within your grasp—and combating the pervasive, often overlooked influence of inflammation on health, in its many forms.**

While the term "inflammation" sounds quite simple, this is actually becoming a major facet of health coming to the forefront of study in many peoples' health struggles all around the globe. It has been mostly overlooked, but now it is being suspected as a contributor to larger diseases, and an important physiological precursor to study in order to understand how these diseases develop.

Inflammation: Both Simple and Complex

When you think of inflammation, you might think of red skin, discomfort, burning sensations, cramps, or other very simple, isolated health problems—problems you can take care of quickly and simply, with nothing too much to worry about.

However, what is being discovered today is that inflammation itself can be at the root of many, many disruptions, ailments, and major diseases. Something so simple-sounding as inflammation, which you might be familiar with in terms of allergies or minor scrapes and injuries, can in fact be an enormous, all-encompassing process in your body that leads to greatly diminished health—and it doesn't limit itself to any one part of the body.

Inflammation can be subtle and unnoticed, but build itself into much bigger problems eventually, if it continues to be ignored. **In this book, I will give you the tools to tackle all kinds of basic inflammation, in its variety of forms: even if it's dealing with something as minor as stomach inflammation, arthritis, or even a headache.** But at the same time, I will equip you with empowering knowledge that could also stave off some of today's most modern and vilified diseases.

Either Way, Why is Inflammation Important?

You might then ask: **"How is inflammation important, and why is it such a big deal?"** Well, this book holds that answer, and it's not a simple one. So with that in mind, I suggest you read on! Throughout these pages we can together dive into all the different ways that inflammation has a role in greater diseases and diminished health.

Again, inflammation might not seem like a huge issue to worry about—but as modern scientific study develops, it is becoming clearer and clearer that inflammation lends itself as the precursor to a number of feared diseases, among them being diabetes, heart disease, arthritis, and even depression.

Further, some of the information in this book might shed a light on some of your own issues: whether or not inflammation is taking hold in your own life, and affecting your own health. But not only that—this book will educate you on how you can navigate, treat, and prevent inflammation on your own, and open up a pathway to many different solutions and approaches, perhaps saving yourself the pricey doctor's visit.

Tips on Inflammation: From My Own Journey

Inflammation invariably causes pain and diminished health, and there are many foods, remedies, and life changes that can help and be explored. I also propone a diet low in gluten, with an emphasis on whole and plant-based foods. Gluten and animal products, science has found, can be a potentially huge contributor to inflammation in the body—and avoiding those foods can be a wise first step in seeing the healing happen.

I myself have had my own struggles with inflammation in my life. My experiences are all contained in this book, the product of my long journey in figuring out what was at the root cause of some of the things I was encountering. A few years ago, I began developing an entire slew of unconnected, but confusing symptoms. Not only did I have digestive upset and frequent headaches, but I also began to develop strange body pains, allergies, and swiftly dwindling energy levels.

Even doctor's visits were not helping, as great as doctors are. I suspected anemia or other things that could be contributing, and yet, blood tests and other examinations showed up with nothing. Confused, I turned to my own careful research and self-empowerment—and when stumbling upon some of the more major studies and health articles on inflammation, something clicked.

Instead of trying to see what I was experiencing as just a simple disease, to "pigeonhole" it and define it, I started to see that what could be happening was a form of systemic inflammation—heightened immune response, as the result of stress, poor eating habits, and other factors.

With an approach to inflammation in mind, I realized that my journey towards better health could be much more simplified. **All this information in hand, I promptly began changing my diet, lifestyle, and seeking the therapies of a number of powerful healing herbs and super foods, all aimed at reducing inflammation.** I switched to a diet without gluten, and a higher value on whole foods, fruits and vegetables, avoiding the consumption of animal products. After a time, amazed, I realized that a lot of these symptoms were slowly beginning to melt away.

Fighting Inflammation: Simple, and there's No Risk!

I was fortunate that inflammation did not contribute to a

bigger issue, and happy that I made the changes I could at the right time. Contained within this valuable book, dear reader, you will find my determined methods of approaching, alleviating, and treating inflammation in your life with an arsenal of foods, herbs, supplements, and lifestyle choices. These simple steps can help boost your health and energy levels, while also preventing the onset of more major diseases like diabetes, heart disease, and even digestive disruption.

I am confident that on some level, the information in this book will point you in the right direction and give you helpful information on how you can change your health for the better, particularly through fighting inflammation. In your hands, you have my journey to use as an empowering example of change—you can take or leave whatever you like, but I am personally certain that you will get something incredible out of this book I've put so much work into!

So let's not waste another moment, and jump straight into the next chapter: **"What is inflammation?"** Without further ado, how about we take a look at inflammation and what it indicates or means in terms of what's happening in our bodies. With an understanding of inflammation as a foundation, we can then delve into the myriad ways we can handle it, which are truly, amazingly simple. Let's get started!

CHAPTER 1

What is Inflammation?

Inflammation is an incredibly common physiological process—and yet, not many might understand or fully know what it means, what it does, and its proper role in the greater scheme of our anatomical rhythms. In this chapter, we'll take a close look at inflammation in all its complexity, as basic a bodily function as it can seem. In my own experience and opinion, the first step to healing is in exactly understanding the functions that need the healing, so you better know how to treat or improve them!

To put it in the simplest terms possible, ***inflammation is the body's way of reacting and responding to harmful influences, foreign invaders, and even tissue breakdown.*** Think of it like your body's "police." Something goes wrong, and inflammation will be there to do the necessary things to preserve and protect.

You might be used to thinking "inflammation is bad." But actually, when you think about its purpose and function, you'll soon realize that inflammation is incredibly good for you—in the right amounts, that is, as inflammation can get out of hand and become damaging.

Inflammation is, in fact, a sign that the body's immune system is activating at the site of threatened health, to remove or cure the cause. When pathogens, illnesses, and bacteria invade—inflammation is triggered to fight any infection. If there is an injury or contusion made up of damaged cells in need of healing, the immune system again triggers inflammation to begin making those damaged cells whole. When foreign objects of any kind—even if they are not disease causing necessarily—enter the body, such as dust or splinters, inflammation happens: like in the case of allergies.

Why? Good question, and the answer is both simple and complex. Inflammation is intended to both protect and heal in any instance, long story short, but the process can be intricate. In the next few sections, we can take a closer look at the actual symptoms of inflammation, and what they actually mean.

Symptoms of Inflammation

You might have observed that in most cases of inflammation, the skin will become reddened—that's because one of the principle organ systems that gets involved is the vascular system. **Skin becoming inflamed and red is a result of blood vessels "vaso-dilating" (opening up) and taking action, pumping as much blood and fluids to the threatened area as possible.**

With this blood comes a wide variety of important immune-related agents to correct the cause: including plasma, T-cells, cytokines, white blood cells, antibodies and finally coagulants, if the inflammation involves bleeding. Other agents will arrive later to begin healing and reconstructing any damaged cells, in the effort to restore any lost function or form.

Redness is one of the most common associations with inflammation, but other symptoms include **pain, swelling, heat, itchiness, and even loss of function.**

Pain resulting from inflammation is caused by the release of chemicals, such as histamine, to alert nerve endings in the injured area of the body: so the body knows to protect and be careful here, as it heals. **Swelling** is usually due to an accumulation of bodily fluids around the site of injury, damage, or infection, as the result of increased plasma and lymphatic action around the site.

Heat is the body pumping warm, basal body temperature-heated blood to the injured site, considered the richest and most active in fighting infection. In the instance of infection, bodily heat can inhibit and even kill certain types of pathogens.

Loss of function inevitably happens if the part of the body in question is damaged or invaded, and even reduced range of motion due to the discomfort of inflammation can occur.

Finally, **itchiness** might happen in less acute and more chronic forms of inflammation, as itchy skin at inflamed sites indicates that the body is striving to heal and shed layers of old skin to make way for the new.

In some forms of inflammation, all of these physiological processes are incredibly noticeable, and even observable at every stage—this is **acute inflammation**. However, **chronic inflammation** takes on a more subtle form, and can be a sign of an unresolved immune response that was never fully healed.

However, what makes these two forms of inflammation truly different—and what are good examples of them?

Acute Inflammation

This form of inflammation might be the one you are most familiar with. Signs of it happening are incredibly obvious and practically immediate after the bodily threat, which typically involves an injury **(cut, burn, sprain, lesion, bruise, splinter)** or the invasion of a bacterial pathogen.

A cut or burn might happen, and promptly, the skin becomes red—the body is immediately on the scene, pumping more blood to this area than usual. Then, it becomes tender, warm and painful, in order to alert the conscious mind and body: "be careful, protect this area!"

Tenderness might enhance pain, as bodily fluids develop around the wound, which is clinically called "edema". If or when bacterial infection sets in on the injury, these symptoms might magnify or worsen, depending on the severity of the injury, or even the specific person's immune health.

As the term "acute" implies, this form of inflammation happens when something sharp or acute occurs. As soon as the source of invasion or injury is removed, the triggers for acute inflammation cease, and the inflammation is resolved.

Whenever you see acute inflammation happening, tell yourself: "This is good inflammation." It means that your body is properly attacking, fighting off, and healing itself from a threat.

What happens, however, when acute inflammation does not resolve itself—or if the body's immune system doesn't know how to properly react? Or, you could ask: **"What are the *bad* forms of inflammation?"**

Chronic Inflammation

Conversely, chronic inflammation can be the other side of the inflammation coin, a much different manifestation from acute—and is the bigger theme and issue to tackle in this book. In terms of its causes and reasons for development, the chronic category is much more complex and less straightforward than its acute counterpart. **One can say that chronic inflammation is a sign of too much inflammation, "overexcited" inflammation, or inflammation going out of control—but then again, it's not always that simple.**

For one, chronic inflammation can result from episodes of acute inflammation, where the pathogen or foreign invader was never successfully or completely removed. But it also might be a symptom or sign of a depleted or disordered immune system, which doesn't know how to properly resolve or complete the inflammation process.

To top it all off, the onset of chronic inflammation can be gradual, delayed and imperceptible, taking as long as months or even years to manifest and observe.

Either way, the body is "stuck" in a cycle of the inflammatory response—for one reason or another, the body gets confused about what it's attacking exactly, and even the cellular nature of what is happening around the sites of invasion can shift into something abnormal and unhealthy.

Instead of a healing process happening in response to an exterior threat, the body begins to simultaneously attack, then heal, then attack itself again. This is, at its most basic, the definition for chronic inflammation—the "bad" inflammation that you want to combat, control, and avoid developing.

While too little inflammation can be dangerous, too much inflammation can be just as undesirable for health. In the case of an acute inflammation situation—if the immune system didn't kick in to fight off infection of foreign invaders, then the site would become overrun with bacteria, necrotize, and rot. Not a pretty picture, I know.

But too much inflammation leads to chronic inflammation, eventually giving way to larger and more serious diseases—such as rheumatoid arthritis, or even cancer. What's worse about chronic inflammation is that it can be sneaky, until it's too late. Awareness of it is important in order for it to not take over your health, and your life.

Low-grade, chronic inflammation and acute inflammation both involve a number of agents, systems, and even organs in the body that play a crucial part in its creation, sustained state, and—eventually—its resolution. Let's look at these next.

The Immune System

The vascular system is a huge part of dealing with acute inflammation, but in chronic inflammation, the immune system tends to grab the wheel and take over. In most forms of chronic inflammatory disorders, abnormalities in the immune system tend to be a common cause—in others, chronic inflammation is instead sourced from other external factors (diet, environment, etc.) and paves the way to serious diseases.

The immune system includes the powers of various antibodies and pathogen-fighting agents in our blood, such as **eicosanoids, leukocytes and cytokines**, which trigger inflammation and immune response. But truly, its complexity extends beyond all that. Mechanisms of coughing, sneezing, crying, urinating, and sweating are all immune responses—expelling mucus and fluids from the body that might contain harmful invading pathogens.

For one reason or another, the immune system can become imbalanced, while its agents and elements become confused about what is a foreign invader—and what is healthy tissue, attacking the wrong one, or both.

Some examples: **"Autoimmune" disorders often feature chronic inflammation as a result of the body attacking itself in certain areas, which is persistent and does not cease unless helped with medication, diet, or lifestyle changes.**

Food allergies are also immune responses that cause the body to attack itself in response to very specific external triggers (i.e. a peanut allergy), which can result in extreme inflammation, discomfort, and at worst, death. Unfortunately, this inflammatory response cannot usually be changed, but it can be treated.

There are a plethora of agents and cells in the body that involve inflammation, but for the sake of brevity, we will only focus on a few. Aspects of the immune system are quite involved with inflammation, some of these helping to determine whether or not chronic inflammation might be present, and even some clues as to how they can be treated.

Mast Cells

These immune cells play a large role in inflammation related to allergies, specifically. **They are central to the effects of asthma, eczema, allergic rhinitis, and whenever you feel "itchy".** Mast cells contain a variety of hormones or "granules," including histamines and cytokines, which contribute to both pain and inflammation. Allergens or other triggers will "cling" to the cell wall of the mast cell, causing it to break and release these hormones—leading to inflammation.

Mast cells also have a part in localized inflammation due to autoimmune disorders, most specifically in the joints. Before histamine or cytokine response happens, a mast cell must be broken by a trigger or allergy. As such, some of the treatments or methods in preventing inflammation from happening, can start with the mast cell.

Histamines

A well-known component of inflammation, histamines tend to be the bigger target when it comes to anti-inflammatory medications, such as anti-histamines. These compounds—technically falling under the category of neurotransmitters—are released by mast cells and proliferate needed pain and inflammation to deal with foreign invaders, as well as helping other immune-active compounds to reach threatened sites via the vascular system.

Histamines are strong aspects of the immune system, and can be commonly involved in chronic inflammatory problems—but they are not the only thing involved!

Histamine reactions produce the typical symptoms of watery eyes, runny nose and a puffy nasal mucus membrane, if there is a trigger that happens within the sinus cavity itself. Elsewhere in the body, histamines are present as typical markers of inflammation—redness, swelling, heat, pain, and reduced function. Interestingly, as a neurotransmitter, histamine serves other uses beyond promoting healing through inflammation:

it plays a role in wakefulness, sleep regulation, and even libido in men.

C-Reactive Proteins

Found in the plasma of the blood, these proteins are found in higher levels when inflammation is present. When testing the body for any detection (especially internal) of inflammation, lab blood tests are often administered to determine **C-reactive protein levels—if above normal, this often indicates low-grade, chronic inflammation is present somewhere in the body.**

High amounts of these proteins are produced in the liver, thus tying in the function of the liver into the larger scope of immune system function and inflammation overall.

The Liver

Modern, biomedical research is beginning to recognize the liver's role in immune function, and hence, inflammation as the result of immune response. Studies show that this major vital organ, not only responsible for allocating and storing important vitamins, minerals and macronutrients, is integral in the health of balancing pro-inflammatory and anti-inflammatory cytokines—the key to maintaining normal levels of inflammation vs. unhealthy ones.

The liver is also holds one of the body's greatest stores of "macrophages," anti-pathogenic

agents that are key instruments of the immune system, often triggered through inflammation. As such, liver health and immune health may be directly related—an unhealthy liver, vis-à-vis with a depleted or disordered immune system, could together be an enormous factor in chronic inflammation or unhealthy inflammatory responses.

As you can tell, there are many functions working together in the body, which take part in inflammation. **The immune system, liver, and countless agents, hormones, and proteins activate dynamically to heal and protect the body in cases of danger— making up the inflammatory response.** In some instances, the body can react quickly and promptly to remove foreign forces; other times, inflammation can become confused and chronic, which can have a destabilizing effect on health when it is supposed to mean well.

But what are the principal causes for inflammation? **What must we look out for and take care of to prevent either acute or chronic inflammation from taking place?** In the next chapter, many different triggers, sources, and causes for inflammation will be explored—all the way from diet and injuries, to lifestyle choices and stress.

CHAPTER 2

What Causes Inflammation?

As important as it is to understand how inflammation works in order to better handle it for your health, so it is vital to know what makes inflammation happen. **No, it's not just foods, injuries and infections that can cause it—there is much, much more.** Before us in this chapter, we'll explore the ins-and-outs of its causes, and what might exactly lead up to those causes happening in turn.

There are a wide variety of influences and triggers that can create this uncomfortable and sometimes persistent symptom. **However, a good way to remember *ANY* potential cause of inflammation is to not forget: inflammation happens as a response to foreign objects, pathogens, agents, or damage to the cells of the body.** It's a way of protecting the body, as unpleasant as it is to experience—and in the end it's a sign of a healthy, robust immune system, if inflammation is incited in the right way.

Just remember: *inflammation protects.* So what can it protect us from, specifically?

Infection and Injury

Most of us will probably associate the process of inflammation with this event above all others. When an injury happens, almost always (naturally,) inflammation ensues. A common range of injuries includes breaks, sprains, cuts, lacerations, and bruises. Of course, however, injuries can be sustained within the body, throughout our vital organs, and may be just as harmful or deadly even if they are not seen.

Whether it's an injury that cuts deep, breaks a bone, or merely bruises the skin—inflammation triggers blood flow to the site of injury, bringing in its wake a plentiful supply of healing immune agents. Cells that have been damaged or destroyed begin to be re-constructed or healed. This is the most common instance where **acute inflammation** occurs.

Sometimes, during the process of injury, bacteria or other pathogens will attempt to invade—causing **infection**. But if inflammation properly sets in, not only is blood staunched and tissue re-construction underway—antibodies like white blood cells flow to the area and prevent infection from spreading. **Inflammation, in fact, is vital in preventing the very worst infections from becoming dangerous!**

Burns

The way the body responds to injuries is very similar to the way it responds to burns, as burns are also injuries, of course. What's different and notable about burns, however, is that the process of acute inflammation can be much more visibly intense and observable—depending on the level or seriousness of the burn.

Same as with injuries, burns involve cellular damage and can also lead to possible infection. However, the immuno-inflammatory response to burns can appear so much more marked, because the cellular damage to the skin does more damage on skin function than some other injuries. **Observing the healing process of a burn is an excellent way to get acquainted with the stages of acute inflammation!**

Common Illnesses and Discomforts

This is the most common form of internal inflammatory response, among the kinds that you cannot see or observe. Sure, injuries and burns can be internal—but most often, when we experience inflammation within the body, it comes as the result of an illness: typically of a bacterial or viral nature.

The common cold, flu, bronchitis, and other frequent illnesses incite the inflammatory and immune response. But many other common discomforts and disruptions can lead to inflammation. **Really, any illness or discomfort caused by the invasion or presence of bacteria, viruses, fungi, parasites, and other pesky pathogens can lead to the inflammatory response.**

Anything from Athlete's Foot, Mononucleosis, and Giardia to Strep Throat, Herpes, or Pinworms creates inflammation to stave off infection, whether that be in the digestive, respiratory, or other bodily systems.

Allergens

In an effort to protect the body, sometimes the immune system responds with inflammation at the wrong times or in greater intensity in proportion to the threat itself. **These "less threatening invaders" are called allergens, whether they be foods, chemicals, or other substances that the body clearly recognizes as "foreign" and not a part of healthy tissues.**

Inflammation can "overreact" to allergens, perceiving them as a threat, when in some cases they are not. They misfire by producing symptoms of inflammation, when there is no real dire cause. This inflammation that the body triggers is commonly called **allergies**, but this is named for responses to foreign objects that are quite intense, and can even result in anaphylaxis or death.

Sensitivities or hypersensitivities are the names for less intense inflammatory responses, such as seasonal allergies or other minor invaders, which can result in uncomfortable inflammation issues (runny nose, puffy sinuses, and irritated stomach). Sometimes, the immune system never fully figures out how to overcome or stop responding to certain allergens, creating the cycle of harmful chronic inflammation.

Poor Diet and Bad Foods

Similar in a way to allergies or sensitivities, these are specifically limited to foods and food choices that can cause irritation of the digestive system. Such foods in this category are often of poor quality, too acidic, or filled with too many processed chemicals or other substances. Stemming from inflammation in the digestive system alone, this immune response can then also spread to other immunologically susceptible parts of the body.

Foods and poor diet can incite the inflammatory response, just as the body can perceive a cut or bruise as a possibility for infection. Being much more similar to an allergy or sensitivity response, however, the body can react harshly to the consumption of poor or inflammatory foods: such as refined sugars, bad fats, or a diet much too high in animal proteins, exactly the same as if those foods were an allergy or sensitivity. Poor diet is another trigger of **chronic inflammation** as a perpetual, debilitating influence on health.

Toxins and Alcohol

Branching out from the inflammatory potential of certain foods, more toxic substances such as drugs or alcohol can further produce a harmful immune response from the body. These can start in the digestive tract as well, and spread outwards to other systems. Whether prescription or recreational, drugs are very hard for the liver to metabolize, along with alcohol.

Drinking too much and taking too many drugs recreationally come with pretty heavy health stigmas to begin with, but some may not know or realize that dependence on their favorite over-the-counter medications or pharmaceuticals—even pills as seemingly harmless as NSAID's—can lead to inflammation, and then even bigger health problems. **Inflammation of the liver** can result, which can then also trigger and influence the rest of the body's immune processes in a very negative, disparaging, and damaging way.

Overexertion and Overuse

Something as simple as overexertion of certain muscles can cause a state of inflammation, which is typically low grade and less acute—**but it can become chronic if healing never properly takes place.** Similar to an injury or allergy situation, where inflammation is activated in the skin or digestive system to help fight off foreign invaders and heal damaged tissues, overexertion is when the muscles are becoming overworked and thus possibly damaged.

Blood pumps to the site of the over-worked muscle, in an effort to re-construct anything that has become damaged due to overuse. Of course, this same inflammatory response can be helpful against potential muscular infection as well. Some slight redness and other inflammation symptoms might be noticed due to muscular overuse, but mostly, symptoms are absent with the exception of noticeable pain, discomfort, and heat. However, you can be rest assured that inflammation is working its due protective processes under the skin, even if you can't see!

Immune System Dysfunction

This root cause of inflammation can be existent in conjunction with, or even as the deeper reason for, other causes. Inflammation itself is considered to be a cut-and-dried immune response, and if the immune system itself is not functioning correctly, then you can expect that inflammation will probably manifest as something out of control or possibly harmful.

Immune system issues, which result in damaging inflammation, can be provoked by too much exposure to allergens, stress, age, obesity, poor diet, or can be acquired from congenital or contracted illnesses. HIV/AIDS, Rheumatoid Arthritis, and Lupus are some examples of illnesses or disorders that have to do with a troubled immune system.

Furthermore, the immune system can either be "underactive" or "depleted," or "overactive" and what is commonly called "autoimmune." In the former, general immune system irregularities might develop, such as an inability to fight off an infection. In the latter, the body literally starts to attack itself, resulting in chronic inflammation and the possibility for greater diseases.

Stress

Emotions can be the gateway to health. **Studies have shown that stress, especially of the chronic kind,**

heightens immune response and sensitivity. Experts at Mayo Clinic state that stress "alters immune system responses and suppresses the digestive system, the reproductive system, and growth processes" as well. Stress literally keys up the body several notches in terms of protecting itself, and thus makes one more likely to experience a misfired inflammatory response—or, even worse, to develop chronic inflammation.

Stress, if intense and prolonged enough, can even change our bodies down to the very genetic level. When someone is exposed to traumatic or anguishing situations for long enough, the body responds by "training" and releasing more macrophages (or immune anti-bodies) that are ready to destroy and fight invaders.

As we both know, of course, being stressed out doesn't mean that there is always something to fight, or an illness invading our good health. But our bodies can't tell that difference. **Even if there is nothing invading or threatening the body physically, stress primes our immune systems to release agents in our blood which are ready to attack at the smallest inconvenience.** It is through these immune changes that chronic inflammation can begin, and start doing its damage.

Knowing how inflammation works, and what causes it, together can lend a clear understanding to the keys to healing it. As you can tell through this chapter, inflammation can come in many, many forms, and influence a vast array of purposes and functions in the body. **In fact, inflammation is known for having its proper place in each of the major systems of our**

physiology, which can also turn unhealthy and cause health problems or illness.

In the next chapter, we'll discover the impact of inflammation—good and bad—in each major organ system of the body. From the digestive and urinary systems, down to the deeper skeletal and muscular ones, inflammation has an important role.

Concerning chronic and misfiring inflammation, however, and as we foray deeper into the world of inflammation overall, a look at each bodily system begs the question: **"Why is it so important to keep certain kinds of inflammation at bay?"**

CHAPTER 3

Why is Minimizing Inflammation Vital to our Overall Health?

This is a good and important question to further our understanding of inflammation, and answering the question "why?" requires a look at the entire body, and at every possible element of its function. In the previous chapters, we studied exactly what inflammation is, what it means in the larger scope of the body's function and even what hormones and compounds it ties in with at the microscopic level. We also looked at the causes that trigger and encourage inflammation to take place.

It's clear that there are proper situations for when inflammation should occur, such as when acute inflammation happens. Then, there are instances when it can become destructive, such as with chronic inflammation. **But really, why is this inflammation bad? What's the worst that can happen if we let inflammation go awry and take its own course?**

Inflammation and the Digestive System

Many influences on health start here in the system regulating nutrition and the foods we eat, which includes our stomach, intestines, colon, and a number of other organs. In fact, a large portion of the list of "causes" from the previous chapter have their biggest impact on the body through this vital system.

Inflammation can start here especially if our diets are terrible, high in inflammatory foods, or full of other substances that have a tendency to irritate the gut. Other factors such as stress, food allergens and immune function can have a hand in inflammation of the digestive system, making it even worse. **So why is inflammation in this system bad especially?**

Well, if the digestive system is inflamed, this can interfere with the proper absorption of essential vitamins, minerals, and macronutrients—and then the body loses health, making it a "double-whammy" blow on the immune system itself. If inflammatory foods and substances go in, along with high stress, chronic and low-grade inflammation can set in—and as long as that inflammation is there, the good foods you can use to reduce inflammation have little to no influence!

This is why minimizing inflammation of the digestive tract is the most important and often first good step of all.

Inflammation and the Heart/Blood Vessels

In terms of inflammation and health, the heart and blood take it the hardest after digestion, bringing it to second place on the list. In fact, some of the leading diseases or causes of illness in the developing world—heart disease, high cholesterol, high blood pressure, diabetes—are by definition illnesses that result from, or cause, chronic inflammation getting out of hand.

Inflammation here can in fact be seen as a "red flag" or warning sign that there could be factors slowly contributing to heart disease or diabetes. Blood vessels, after all, transport the majority of the substances and foods our bodies consume through the digestive system. As such, poor diet and food choices create inflammation here as well—such as in the case of high bad cholesterols clogging the arteries.

The worst consequence to an inflamed vascular system can lead to heart attacks, bodily damage due to poor circulation, and even cancer; this makes minimizing inflammation of the heart and blood vessels an integral health priority.

Inflammation and the Respiratory System

Most might overlook this system as playing a role in chronic inflammation. Sure, acute inflammatory responses happen here sometimes, like with allergies, bronchitis, infections, and the common cold. But we think that anything that impacts the lungs and airways comes and goes quickly. **This is not true—and in fact, inflammation of the lungs and airways can be huge forewarnings of dangerous inflammation in the body, even cancer.**

Before you get uneasy about your own respiratory health, remember that cancer or lung disease is really at the most extreme end of the spectrum. Most inflammations of the respiratory system are signs of acute inflammations healing themselves in time. Still, symptoms like coughing, hacking, wheezing, and excessive phlegm can be signs of present inflammation and even some immune disorder—a warning of something more major.

Inflammation and the Urinary System

The urinary system is often understated, but as it involves waste output and the kidneys themselves—a vital organ—this system is nonetheless incredibly important to take into account. To top it all off, there is a large potential for inflammation to happen in the kidneys and urinal waterways that simply should not be overlooked!

Inflammation here can be either acute or chronic, and sourced either from dietary choices, toxins, and yes, autoimmune disorders. **What's important to realize, too, about dysfunction in urine output is that when it's not working correctly, blood can leak into the urine—and then flush out a large amount of helpful antibodies and immune agents from the system.**

Inflammation in the urinary system, much like with the digestive system, should be minimized in order to help the body reach healthy balance and stability.

Inflammation and the Skeletal System

Inflammatory diseases that afflict the bones are among the highest-occurring in the developing world. The leading inflammatory disorders of the skeletal system are **osteoarthritis** and **rheumatoid arthritis**, both of which are triggered by depletion or dysfunction of cartilage and joint lubrication—and thus causing inflammation and pain in the bones and joints themselves.

Truly, arthritis of both types can be debilitating if not crippling, but inflammation in the skeletal system at its very worst tends to only create a high potential for pain and discomfort. **Still, minimizing inflammation in this system is important to living a comfortable and mobile life, even if it doesn't pave the way to a worse disease**.

Furthermore, in the case of rheumatoid arthritis (an autoimmune disease), chronic inflammation of the skeletal system can be a marker for larger sources of inflammation elsewhere in the body, especially of an immune-based nature—which should become a goal to reduce for better health.

Inflammation and the Muscular System

Much like the skeletal system, muscular inflammation (also called **"myositis"**) is more of a marker or signal that there could be chronic inflammation present somewhere else in the body. Minimizing inflammation in this system is mostly important in terms of living a comfortable, mobile life, but also preventing the possibility for greater disease. Most of the time, however, muscular inflammation is the result of an isolated injury undergoing acute inflammation, and with some medical intervention it resolves itself with time.

However, in some cases, inflammation of the muscles is the sign of an auto-immune disorder: the body's protective system dysfunctions and starts attacking the body's muscle. Sometimes, these disorders can be linked to larger diseases in the body, such as cancer. For that reason, the muscular system is still an important facet to watch out for with inflammation!

Inflammation and the Nervous System

Some might forget that the nervous system can fall prey to inflammation, just like other systems can. This facet of the functioning body can be the most complex and far-reaching of all, thus making inflammation in its quarter sometimes the most difficult to understand, pinpoint, or even study. But it's true—inflammation, both chronic and acute, can take a hold of the brain and nerves.

Recent studies are showing, for example, that low-grade inflammation of the brain can be a trigger for depression, or even that depression and stress itself can lead to inflammation. Posted in a recent article by Medical News Today, research in Canada underwent a thorough imaging scan of the brains of 40 different people—half with varying forms of depression, half without. In those with depression, inflammation around the brain was greater than normal by up to 30%, and higher on that scale for those with more severe forms especially.

Either one leads to the other, and data shows that this is mostly uncertain—but what's most important to realize is that inflammation, even on a chronic and low-grade level, can have a pivotal impact on one's way of life through our consciousness and thinking, making it important to minimize here too.

Inflammation and the Immune System

While we both know that inflammation is in and of itself a function of the immune system, it can be believed that the immune system itself can become "inflamed."

This is an excellent way to understand the state of "autoimmune" disorders, or when the immune system is too "over stimulated" and begins to attack completely harmless and healthy areas of the body. **If one can view the immune system as a separate organ in the need of some anti-inflammatory therapy, this can then have a far-reaching, anti-inflammatory repercussion on all the other affected systems of the body.**

As it goes according to the "holistic" model of health (i.e., treating the whole body, not just the sum of its parts), in order to best treat a disorder, one most go to the root of the cause or study the whole picture. Hence, in terms of treating inflammation system-by-system, **one must make sure that they are being proactive about treating the immune system itself too—not just the isolated areas where chronic inflammation is being experienced.**

Now we have a sufficient understanding of inflammation as it manifests throughout the body, and why it's important to keep it under control—in cases of chronic inflammation—to improve health on all levels.

Next, as we move into the following chapter, let's take a look at the actual diseases that involve inflammation, as well as more major illnesses and diseases inflammation itself can lead up to. Just like this chapter we walked through, ailments resulting from inflammation can spring up in practically any system of the body—some can be minor, while others more damaging.

CHAPTER 4

Conditions and Illnesses Related to Inflammation

Inflammation is an incredibly common function we encounter in health, time and time again. **It's involved in some of the most well-known illnesses and disorders we talk about and deal with every day, while at the same time, it has an influential presence in some illnesses we may not readily realize.** It can take part in maladies that are incredibly minor and almost harmless, if we take care of them and treat them well enough.

But, as this book reveals, inflammation can also push our health downwards towards some of the most major and feared diseases of the day. For that very reason, an understanding of the conditions and diseases involved is absolutely crucial for optimum, low-inflammatory health.

Which brings us to our next discussion about inflammation: **"What conditions and illnesses involve inflammation?"** Which ailments do we really have to worry about in managing chronic inflammation? It's just as important to know the "end-road" for inflammatory mishaps, as it is to know how it works and what causes it.

So, without further ado, let's delve into the potential

illnesses and conditions inflammation can lead us towards. As we outlined previously, such maladies can emerge in practically any organ system of the body—and for that reason, the more possibilities we can explore and prepare ourselves healthfully for, the better.

But, first things first, let me give you an amazing tip on how to determine whether or not a common condition or ailment has to do with inflammation!

The Meaning of the Suffix "-itis"

You've probably heard of "colitis," "gastritis," or "rhinitis?" Try "contact dermatitis," or "bronchitis."

Did you ever realize that any sort of health condition that ends with –itis means that it involves inflammation? With dermatitis, for example, "derma-" is a Latin prefix meaning "skin." The suffix –itis means "inflammation," literally. Push them together, and you've got "inflammation of the skin." Easy to put it together, right?

Therefore, in order to know whether a disease involves inflammation, all you've got to do is brush up on your Latin, or dust off that old medical terminology book.

If you go to the doctor's office, or suspect you've got something inflammatory going on with your health, keep your ears perked for the word "-itis." You'll know that inflammation is at play, and that it's time to go home and do some research—and particularly determine if this is a type of inflammation you have to keep an eye on. Paired with the wonderful advice of your doctor, of course, knowledge of inflammatory illnesses is power.

However, do be forewarned—just because a disease name doesn't include "-itis," doesn't mean that it does not involve inflammation at all. Research, gain knowledge, and empower your own education on the subject of any illness and whether or not it involves inflammation. So far, you're lucky—the following section will be an enormously helpful tool in getting started, and knowing the "what's what" with inflammation.

Minor Ailments Related to Inflammation

The following are only minor and relatively common conditions that either give rise to inflammation, or are created by it. Many of these are able to be treated at home, with home remedies, healthful foods and healing herbs.

Acne. Some kinds of acne are inflammatory, while others are not. Hair follicles in the skin can become blocked by dead skin or bacteria, resulting in inflammation.

Allergies (Rhinitis). Mucus membranes in the nasal passages become enflamed by foreign objects—puffy eyes, nose, and "runniness" is the body's inflammatory response, which directly reflects the immune system's "relationship" with that allergen.

Bronchitis. With potential to become a more serious condition, this involves inflammation of the bronchial tubes, typically accompanying or caused by an infection.

Chronic Fatigue. A complex condition, chronic fatigue might be involved with low-grade chronic inflammation all throughout the body, due to an overwhelmed and stressed out immune system.

U.T.I.s (Cystitis). Characterized by inflammation of the bladder, this condition tends to be noticeably caused or worsened by stress, and triggered by infection.

Viral Infections/Colds. Not quite classically "inflammatory," but the cough, runny nose, and sore throat of this common illness is very much an immune response, and can reflect inflammatory/immune health!

Eczema/Dermatitis. Inflammation of the skin that can either be chronic (eczema) or acute (contact dermatitis). Simple to treat with home remedies and herbs, and helps convey immune health to some extent.

Food Hypersensitivities. Mild to moderate immune reaction to certain foods, which creates inflammation and irritation of the digestive tract. Can be directly related to a struggling immune system.

Stomach Upset (Gastritis). This involves inflammation of the stomach lining, which can either be acute or chronic, caused by either stress, food, or immune issues.

Gout. A diet-induced inflammation of the joints, caused by high build-up of "uric acid"—a protein by-product. Painful, but manageable with foods and herbs.

Headaches. Most headaches are caused by some inflammation, especially the most common headaches: sinus headaches, which can be involved with sinusitis. Increase in occurrence and likelihood of headaches can be related to chronic inflammation.

Muscular Inflammation (Myositis). Most muscular inflammation is caused by overexertion/overuse, although the actual term "myositis" indicates that there is often immune dysfunction involved—and thus, a misfiring of chronic inflammation.

Pneumonia. With the potential to become something more serious, like bronchitis, this involves infection and inflammation of the lungs—but with fluid that fills the lungs, thus making this illness need special attention and treatment.

Psoriasis. Irregular inflammation of the skin, involving an abnormal immune response to healthy human skin cells. Some studies show a connection between psoriasis and liver health—with the liver being considered a large immune factor in modern research. As stated by the National Psoriasis Foundation on recent findings, "researchers found that people with psoriasis were still approximately 70% more likely to have Non-Alcoholic Fatty Liver Disease," which directly links psoriasis to an unhealthy liver and immune function.

Sinusitis. When the sinus cavity becomes inflamed, this can result in headaches, coughs, and facial pain. It can be caused by bacterial or viral infection, or even allergies—those with "seasonal allergies" and frequent sinusitis might have a more sensitive immune system, and thus inflammatory response.

Major Illnesses Related to Inflammation

Below are listed the more major complications that arise from inflammation. Most of these can be helped or managed some with food or diet, but often times, the need of a professional healthcare provider is absolutely necessary—as some of these conditions can become very damaging, or potentially life threatening.

Arthritis (Rheumatoid/Osteo). Painful and debilitating inflammation of the joints. Rheumatoid is the result of an autoimmune dysfunction that attacks joint-protective cartilage, while Osteo is due to overexertion, nutritional deficiency, or depletion of synovial fluid—both arthritis types involve inflammation.

Alzheimer's. This psychological disease, resulting in memory loss and dementia, is under intense study nowadays with evidence showing that chronic inflammation could be one of its major precursors.

Asthma. A chronic inflammatory response that can shut down and obstruct airways, which can be life threatening. A combination of genetics, stress levels, immune strength, and possible allergens can contribute.

Cancer. Chronic inflammation has long been studied and connected with cancer development, thus in part making cancer considered partially an inflammatory disease.

Celiac Disease. A severe, genetic, autoimmune and inflammatory response to wheat, rye, and other grains containing gluten, which occurs in the intestines. Celiac's, when untreated, can end with severe anemia and digestive issues.

Crohn's Disease. An autoimmune, inflammatory disorder of the intestines, which often creates symptoms similar to IBS/IBD (Inflammatory Bowel Diseases). Can often be triggered by poor food and diet choices.

Depression. Studies reveal a connection between depression and inflammation—either that low-grade inflammation can lead to the disorder, or vice versa, with inflammation occurring in and around the brain. Chair of Canadian research on Depression, Dr. Jeffrey Myer, states "Depression is a complex illness... but we now believe that inflammation in the brain is one of these changes, and that's an important step forward."

Diabetes. Inflammation has also been shown through recent research to have a huge role in diabetes: the body's inability to properly process sugars can also release pro-inflammatory cytokines. This inflammation plays a part in the destructive circulatory issues inherent in diabetes, which most often results from a combination of genetics and poor diet choices. One Spanish biomedical study specifically states that "clinical studies have generated evidence that fibromyalgia is associated with immune dysregulation of circulatory levels of pro-inflammatory cytokines, affecting the neural dysfunction of pain-related neurotransmitters."

Fibromyalgia. Studies reveal that fibromyalgia, a complex and mysterious disorder to diagnose, may be related to an increase of pro-inflammatory cytokines in the body—causing fatigue and pain all over the body.

Food Allergies. More intense than food hypersensitivities, food allergies (i.e. peanut, nightshade) involve a more intense immune response, which can even involve anaphylaxis and sometimes, death.

Hashimoto's Thyroiditis. An autoimmune disorder, where inflammatory antibodies attack the thyroid—thus creating an autoimmune form of hypothyroidism. The thyroid regulates metabolism and hormone dispersal, which can make this inflammation-oriented disorder result in weight gain and fatigue.

Heart Attack/Congestive Heart Failure. Arterial build up, due to poor diet or inflammatory foods, can lead to serious heart complications. Inflammation of the arteries is often a marker of possible heart disease, which can result in heart attack and even death.

Inflammatory Bowel Disease (IBS/IBD). A generalized disorder, this characterizes inflammation all over the digestive tract, due to a number of possible influences—common symptoms being alternating constipation and diarrhea.

Lupus. A group of severe autoimmune, inflammatory diseases that can afflict the kidneys, liver, skin, heart and lungs through over-stimulated, damaging chronic inflammation—with photosensitivity being a common symptom.

Multiple Sclerosis. An inflammatory disease where the nerve endings, spinal cord, and brain are damaged by a progressive destruction of the immune system.

Inflammation arises in an enormous range of conditions and illnesses. Now, it's time for us to take a look at the most exciting aspects of healing inflammation itself, beyond just understanding it—**through foods, diet, lifestyle choices, and healing herbs!**

CHAPTER 5

How Can I Avoid and Heal Inflammation?

Now we're delving into the chapter we've all been waiting for: healing inflammation itself. We've started out with a both broad and deep understanding of inflammation, how it works, what causes it and how you can expect it to manifest. Now, it's time to move on to the part where you can take some control!

As we've discussed, inflammation can arise in many different body systems. It can be triggered by a wide variety of causes or influences, and be helpful in some instances while harmful in others, especially if it becomes chronic and low-grade. It can create or take part in minor ailments to major illnesses, some of which we can manage at home; others, we must seek professional help for its seriousness.

But here's the thing: inflammation, whether part of a major or minor disorder, can always be managed with your own choices. Inflammation can be part of a disease, or it might not be. Either way, no matter what you are undergoing, there is no harm in managing inflammation affecting your health in your own way.

Inflammation is part of many diseases, but remember, it is also a way that your immune system expresses itself. There is no harm that can possibly be done in fighting chronic inflammation or healing your own immune system, especially if you are selecting natural, safe, whole foods, supplements, and herbs—and making empowering life choices, to boot! **In this final chapter, let's take a look at all the many different ways you can boost your immune health and keep inflammation at bay.**

Foods to Avoid

Sometimes, it's easier to ask "what should I *not* eat?" instead of what you should eat—at least, for some. A good deal of foods can possibly trigger and escalate the inflammatory response of the body, all the way from allergies to—yes, even cancer, some studies show.

Peruse the following list, and then stick to it if you're wishing to fight inflammation!

Animal Proteins. Studies are mounting that a diet higher in animal foods, versus plant based ones, is comparable nutritionally—except that the animal foods caused more inflammation in those who consumed consistent amounts. Dairy in particular is acid forming and a common dietary allergen, known to promote long-term inflammation in the body.

To reduce inflammation, consider lowering the amount of animal proteins you eat, or omitting them from your diet altogether. These include any kind of meat or seafood, but also milk, cheese, yogurt, eggs and poultry. A study by the Proceedings of the National Academy of Sciences found a certain sugar in red meat specifically called "Neu5Gc", which was observed to increase the likelihood of tumor development and carcinoma in non-carnivorous animals—humans being one example.

In regards to arthritic inflammation, Dr. John McDougall states that a healthy, plant based diet "supplies antioxidants and other phytochemicals that keep the joints strong and repair damage. Animal studies have shown that the foods consumed on the rich American diet fail to provide adequate antioxidants to destroy the damaging free radicals that form in the joint tissues."

Corn Syrups (and High Fructose Corn Syrup). This processed syrup is added for thickness and sweetening to many processed foods, but studies prove its pro-inflammatory and harmful effects, even pushing some who eat high amounts of it towards insulin problems and then to diabetes. Avoid foods with corn syrup, especially high fructose corn syrups.

One study by the American Society of Nephrology found that fructose, not in its whole form (refined and without the natural fiber normally found in fruit) "induces inflammatory changes in vascular cells, at physiologic concentrations." The study then goes on to state that chronic inflammation is commonly observed in metabolic syndromes, which then lead to hypertension—raised blood pressure, which then increases the likelihood of heart disease and stroke.

Processed Foods in general. Besides corn syrups, there are a wide variety of inflammatory chemicals, preservatives, and substances added to foods that increase inflammation. Some of these can be hydrogenated oils, palm kernel oils, MSG, food dyes, and practically anything ending in –ate means it's a non-natural preservative.

Stay away from these! Some examples include fast food, sodas, and pretty much any food in which you study the ingredients—and it mostly includes an enormous paragraph of huge, wordy chemical-sounding things that you don't know what they mean.

Fried Foods (especially deep fried!). Those lovely potato chips, French fries, donuts, and chicken-fried steaks you love to much on are terrible for inflammation. Many of the oils used to deep-fry (or even lightly fry) most purchasable foods are filled with trans-fats—the worst fats you can eat, and the ones most infamous for clogging your arteries.

Enriched, bleached, white and refined flours. Keep an eye on gluten products in general, of which flour-based products are full of. Flours of these categories, especially, are filled with enrichments, excipients, and additives that irritate the intestinal lining—which then promote bodily inflammation.

On the gluten subject, flours made from wheat, rye, kamut, or possibly oats as well contain gluten, which—regardless if you have a gluten sensitivity, Celiac's, or not—have a role in creating some irritation to some degree of your digestive tract. Consider a diet that omits gluten completely, or at the very least, minimizes it. **Stay away from processed baked goods especially, such as donuts, cakes, bagels and croissants.** These also tend to be chock-full of trans fats.

Bad fats. These include trans fats and saturated fats, the latter being a type of fat often found in animal products such as meat, dairy and eggs. Enough said—avoid the bad fats and focus on the good, whole-food ones, such as nuts, seeds and avocados.

Refined sugars. Not only is it good to opt for more natural sweeteners, such as pure maple syrup, raw sugar, coconut sugar or stevia, but it is also good to reduce your consumption of any refined sugar overall. **Refined sugar can increase inflammation in the body—and can worsen symptoms of inflammatory and auto-immune diseases like arthritis, diabetes, and vascular disease.**

Reduce refined sugars but do not decrease the consumption of whole-food sugars such as fruits and root vegetables. Furthermore—be a sugar watchdog when studying the ingredients in your food. Anything in the ingredients ending in –ose (fructose, glucose) is a refined sugar.

Foods to Emphasize

After formulating a list of what not to eat, a good next step is to focus on what you should. The wonderful thing about bad versus good foods, and with inflammation specifically, is that there are plenty of foods to choose from out there that don't promote inflammation whatsoever.

Sure, they might not be your favorite midnight munchie,

or include the ice cream of your favorite flavor. It's also incredibly hard when the mainstream diet of the developed world is mostly inflammatory, filled with processed foods and junk. But focusing on an anti-inflammatory diet just takes a little willpower, and a deep realization that there are a lot of anti-inflammatory foods out there.

Here is a list of your greatest, chronic-inflammation food fighters out there.

Foods High in Omega-3 Fatty Acids. You can find these in high amounts in a lot of seafood, but because fish does not play a protective role in inflammation, I emphasize a path with plant-based sources. Try flaxseed, walnuts, almonds, olives, coconut products and a variety of other nuts to fill your dietary needs.

Studies have shown that inflammation in the body can be curbed incredibly well by increasing sources of these long-strain, polyunsaturated fatty-acids. As disclosed by a 2008 finding by the Department of Medicine in Massachusetts, along with the Harvard Medical School: "Polyunsaturated fatty acids (omega-6 and omega-3 fatty acids)... play an important role in regulation of inflammation. Generally, omega-6 fatty acids promote inflammation, whereas omega-3 fatty acids have anti-inflammatory properties."

Foods High in Antioxidants. Studies highly support the addition of antioxidants in the diet, which demonstrate notable influence on suppressing harmful immune activity—specifically chronic inflammation. Antioxidants can be found in a wide variety of plant-based foods, and even herbs. The Institute of Nutrition in the UK declares that a wide variety of antioxidant nutrients have exhibited anti-inflammatory action against symptoms of inflammatory diseases, such as arthritis, pancreatitis, and even HIV and AIDS.

Some good examples: green kale, broccoli, purple potatoes, cabbage, blueberries, raspberries, blackberries, cherries, red/black/pinto beans, apples, and yes—in moderation—dark chocolate (dairy free).

Foods High in Fiber. The root of inflammation starts with the foods we eat and the digestive system. One of the best ways you can keep your digestive tract running smoothly and inflammation-free, is to ensure that your diet is high in fiber.

Fiber is found in a wide range of plant products, and is a vital and natural part of the human diet in reducing inflammation and even toxicity that can build up. Foods that are high in fiber include **legumes** (such as lentils, chickpeas and beans), and an array of **fruits, root vegetables and vegetables**, especially leafy greens.

Complex carbohydrates made up of **gluten-free grains** are another amazing source of fiber, such as quinoa, amaranth, sorghum and buckwheat.

Foods that Boast Anti-Inflammatory Effects. Beyond fiber, Omega-3's and antioxidants, some foods are developing a well-known reputation for fighting and reducing chronic inflammation.

One of these categories of foods is the **Brassicaceae**

family of vegetables, which includes kales, cabbage, radishes, turnips, mustard greens, and cauliflower, just to name a few. Studies by the Tokyo University of Science showed that a compound found in most Brassicas called sulforaphane was observed as having the best anti-inflammatory effects, with **broccoli** having the highest levels of the compound. Extracts of the plant were so powerful, they even prevented worsening inflammation in stomach ulcers.

Furthermore, the **Allium** family of vegetables showed a sulphur-based compound that helped modulate the immune system in many studies. The Alliums include leeks, garlic, onions, scallions, chives and shallots.

Foods that are WHOLE, Hormone, Pesticide, Herbicide, and Additive Free. That's a lot of words to describe something so simple, but it says a lot. A focus on finding plant foods from sources as natural and organic as possible is not a high priority for some, but who knows what chemicals sprayed on your food can do to you, especially if it is designed to kill insects and other plants? If even food additives can cause inflammation, then it's likely that a spray or herbicide will probably do the same.

For that reason, it's a safer bet that buying organic foods will help you go the distance in reducing inflammation. Studies on arthritis patients, who regularly suffer from inflammation, show that diets focused on whole, organic, and naturally grown foods have more to show for themselves than watered down, conventional foods. Dr. Christine G. Parks, at the National Institute of Environmental Health Sciences in America, led a study that confirmed in increased likelihood of contracting auto-immune diseases when exposed to pesticides.

So, in purchasing your fruits, veggies, nuts, legumes and grains—try sticking to organic where possible.

Spice it up. Herbs and spices have some of the most powerful antioxidant effects, but which ones boast the best anti-inflammatory benefits? Studies have shown that the following herbs and spices prove most effective in reducing inflammation in the body: **cloves, ginger, rosemary and turmeric.** Consider regularly spicing up your daily meals with these healthful additions, all of which mimic effects similar to anti-inflammatory drugs without the side effects. You can also brew your chosen spices and enjoy as an antioxidant rich, inflammatory fighting tea.

Other beneficial anti-inflammatory herbs and spices include: **black pepper, chamomile, cardamom, cilantro (coriander), basil, cinnamon, garlic, fennel seeds, parsley and nutmeg.**

Herbal Healing, Supplements and Lifestyle/Diet Tips for Inflammatory Conditions

Supplements and herbs of many kinds are becoming popular these days, but have also been used anciently to heal a wide variety of disorders. **Furthermore, the amount of anti-inflammatory herbs and natural**

medicines out there in the world seem almost endless, once you get started studying them!

As we delve into the natural healing world of inflammation, we'll take a look at the most common and major specific conditions which involve this immune response, like we did in Chapter 4—but categorize the healing methods for each inflammatory disorder by bodily system, similar to Chapter 3.

Step-by-step, and in as thorough a manner as possible, home-healing for most every inflammatory disease will be approached—whether it involves herbs, supplements, and small lifestyle and diet tips to reduce unhealthy levels of chronic, harmful inflammation.

Digestive System: Natural Relief Techniques

Food hypersensitivities are a minor inflammatory condition we've discussed, while **Celiac Disease, Crohn's Disease, Food Allergies,** and **Inflammatory Bowel Disease** are the more major manifestations of inflammation in the digestive system. Through eating the wrong foods and being exposed to too many allergens, these conditions can develop, or the inflammation related to them can be made even worse.

Not to fear: there are a number of herbs, supplements, and other tips that can help with the inflammation of the gut directly.

Herbs:
Ginger (Zingiber officinale) for mild troubles like simple stomach upset; **Goldenseal (Hydrastis canadensis)**, used as an anti-inflammatory, antibiotic, and digestive tonic for hundreds of years; immuno-modulating medicinal mushrooms, like **Reishi (Ganoderma spp.)** have been shown to help the immune system "normalize," which can be helpful for digestive allergies or immune issues, like Crohn's. There are an incredible amount of supporting studies of Reishi in Chinese Pharmacological medicine trials, one of which concludes "Reishi increases numbers and functions of virtually all cell lines in the immune system, such as natural killer cells, antibody-producing B cells, and the T cells responsible for rapid response to a new or 'remembered' antigen."

Supplements:
Omega-3 supplements are common in helping ease digestive inflammation. For best results, opt for plant-based sources such as **Evening Primrose Oil** or even pure **GLA (Gamma Linoleic Acid)**. **Selenium, Zinc,** and **Calcium** are common mineral supplements that help regulate digestion inflammation.

Lifestyle Tips:
Eat foods high in fiber and often for minimizing digestive inflammation. Avoid over use of prescription pills, drugs, or alcohol—which worsen digestive inflammation directly. Overall, focus on a good diet absolutely necessary, and reducing stress and anxiety in lifestyle, which can contribute to digestive abnormalities.

Vascular System (Heart and Blood): Natural Relief Techniques

Diabetes and **heart disease** are two of the leading causes of death and illness in the developing world, both of which involve the buildup of chronic, systemic inflammation. The following methods are ways you can help manage this brand of inflammation in your own life, while seeking the professional help of your licensed care provider to take care of the more major aspect of these potentially life-threatening diseases.

Herbs:
Hawthorn (Cretaegus monogyna) is hailed both in conventional and natural medicine for its heart-strengthening effects, which can be an aid to heart disease. **Cayenne Pepper (Capsicum anuum)** is a traditional blood-tonic that studies are showing can prevent the likelihood of heart attack. The American Nutrition Association states; "Research from the University of Cincinnati shows that a common, over-the-counter pain salve (made of capsaicin, the active constituent in Cayenne) rubbed on the skin during a heart attack could serve as a cardiac-protectant, preventing or reducing damage to the heart while interventions are administered."

Supplements:
Fiber supplements may be added for a heart-healthy diet and reducing inflammation, as it helps cut cholesterol levels. **Stanols** and **Sterols** are also commonly prescribed, which are naturally found in nuts, but

can be taken as supplements. **Coenzyme-q10** is a naturally-occurring human enzyme that can be taken as a supplement, which naturally helps lower blood pressure.

Lifestyle Tips:
Exercise is important, especially aerobic, to maintain heart health and to prevent heart disease: such as light jogging or swimming (take care not to over-exert yourself). Reducing stress can also help, not only with lowering the immune response of inflammation, but it can aid with lowering blood pressure—as high blood pressure increases the likelihood of heart attack.

Respiratory System: Natural Relief Techniques

Allergies, common colds, and a wide variety of other inflammatory conditions can arise in the lungs and air passages. **Bronchitis** and **pneumonia** enter the realm of more serious conditions, while **asthma** can be one of the more major respiratory and inflammatory illnesses that inhibit ways of life. Luckily, there are also a range of herbs, supplements, and lifestyle tips that can help on this level.

Herbs:
Both Echinacea (Echinacea spp.) and **Goldenseal (Hydrastis canadensis)** are highly popular and studied intensely for their antibiotic, anti-inflammatory influences on upper respiratory conditions. One review of Echinacea in 1999 by the Journal of Family Practice overlooked 8 studies of the plant, all of which

showed strong evidence of shortening the duration of colds as a treatment. Herbs containing **thujone**, like **Cedar (Thuja occidentalis)**, **Yarrow (Achillea millefolium)**, and **Sage (Salvia officinalis)** have been studied for their anti-asthmatic effects, with good success.

Supplements:

Vitamin C and **Zinc** supplements can be prescribed for respiratory health. Pills of **N-Acetyl Cysteine** are commonly used by some for allergies, bronchitis, and even lung cancer —with it being a prominent antioxidant, in supplement form it no doubt lends its support against oxidative stress, which compounds the inflammatory response.

Lifestyle Tips:

Avoid smoking tobacco and other substances, which can promote inflammation of the respiratory tract. Furthermore, it can be a real immune stress on the lungs working in environments high in toxins, chemicals, and pollutants that can be inhaled. Exercise is thought to be beneficial to lung health if possible, especially aerobic exercise like jogging or swimming.

Skeletal System: Natural Relief Techniques

Rheumatoid Arthritis, Osteoarthritis, and **Gout** are the major disorders of the bones that can cause inflammation. Many herbs, supplements, and lifestyle choices have been set in place—especially since these disorders, to some extent largely immune-based, involve quite a bit of inflammation.

Herbs:
Ginger (Zingiber officinale) and **Turmeric (Curcuma longa)** are quickly becoming studied and praised herbs for helping with the painful inflammation of all arthritis types, through the activity of their active constituent *curcumin*. For Rheumatoid types, medicinal mushrooms like **Cordyceps (Cordyceps spp.)** can help modulate the self-attacking autoimmune element, with one Korean study finding that "Cordyceps extract increased pro-inflammatory cytokines through the activation of NF-KB, further suggesting that it may prove useful as an immune-enhancing agent in the treatment of immunological disease." For Gout, herbs like **Cedar (Thuja officinalis)** and **Stinging Nettle (Urtica dioica)** are favored for helping pass the uric acid crystals created by gout.

Supplements:
Omega-3 supplements are often prescribed for any arthritis to reduce the body's reaction to inflammation. **Calcium** and **Vitamin D3** are given especially in cases of osteoarthritis to help rebuild cartilage and damaged bone.

Lifestyle Tips:
Many regimens for arthritis heavily encourage exercise as part of the plan, which has been proven to show relief of inflammatory pain—but also, for patients to lose weight, if weight problems are contributing to the problem. Diet comes in at a tie: avoiding inflammatory foods and eating a good diet high in whole fruits and vegetables, with plenty of Omega-3's, is vital to soothing inflammation in all types of arthritis.

The Nervous System: Natural Relief Techniques

It can be as simple as a transient headache, all the way through to clinical depression, Alzheimer's disease or Multiple Sclerosis (MS). It's apparent that inflammation does have a role in the organ system of our bodies that rules consciousness, feelings, and the way we think. Herbs, supplements, and some lifestyle tips do provide some opportunities for relief, studies and empirical knowledge have shown.

Herbs:

Feverfew (Tanacetum matricaria) has shown efficacy in trials with helping headaches of an inflammatory nature—sinus headaches, and even the onset of migraines. **St. John's Wort (Hypericum perforatum)** holds immense respect in the herbal world for helping with mild depressions, perhaps even the inflammation aspect, while studies are mounting around the medicinal mushroom **Lion's Mane (Hericium erinaceus)** showing promise for the healing and recovery of Alzheimer's and MS sufferers.

One study of the mushroom by the Fungal Biotechnology Lab in Kuala Lumpur, Malaysia, states: "Hericenones and erinacines isolated from the medicinal mushroom Hericium erinaceus can induce nerve growth factor synthesis in nerve cells," which is essential for the maintenance of major brain functions.

Supplements:
5-HTP and Melatonin are common supplements for depression, headaches and Alzheimer's, and might have a slight anti-inflammatory effect, though unknown. Caffeine in supplement form has shown very effective for headaches, while the B Vitamins and minerals Riboflavin and Magnesium are often prescribed to those who commonly experience headaches of an inflammatory nature, or depression. For MS, vitamin D has been surmised to be the most helpful supplement for the condition.

Lifestyle Tips:
For mental and nervous issues, decreasing and reducing stress or depression factors in one's life can be key. Exercise has also shown very effective for nervous disorders, especially depression, and getting regular, quality sleep is important to maintain for good mental health and strong nerves. Some headaches might depend on a matter of maintaining a good diet that avoids inflammatory foods.

The Immune System: Natural Relief Techniques

At the root of it all lies the immune system itself, responsible for all triggers of inflammation anywhere in the body. **Chronic Fatigue** and **Fibromyalgia** are milder but nevertheless life-altering disorders presupposed to be of inflammatory, immune origin—while **Lupus** is a common immune disorder that has strong, proven connections to immune health, but which can manifest anywhere in the body. Today, there are a number of ways to manage these matters with natural remedies.

Herbs:

The world of herbal healing is wide open in terms of immune-enhancing and modulating remedies. Medicinal mushrooms like **Chaga (Inonotus obliquus)** have shown potential in halting immune dysfunction, while empowering immune in correct ways for correct inflammatory response, especially in the development of cancer. Says one Polish study by the Department of Medical Biology, "Chaga... elicited anticancer effects which were attributed to decreased tumor cell proliferation... Of note is the fact that it produced no or low toxicity in tested normal cells. The data presented could open interesting paths for further investigations (of Chaga) as a potential anticancer agent."

Licorice root (Glycyrrhiza glabra) is another popular and well-documented plant that can help regulate the immune system at its roots, for some. Studies seem to support its activity especially against viral threats, with one by the *Microbiology* and *Immunology* journal observing licorice boosting interferon levels in the body, which is the system's natural antibody against viruses.

Supplements:

All vitamins and minerals as a supplement are believed to be important to immune function, so all are recommended. Those with immune dysfunction might specifically be prescribed **selenium, B Vitamins, Vitamin E** and **Vitamin C**, however.

Lifestyle Tips:
Those wishing to improve immune health get advice all across the board: eat well, eat fruits and vegetables, avoid inflammatory foods, get enough exercise, reduce stress, and even form good relationships! It's clear that emotional well-being and healthy inflammation levels go hand-in-hand.

Make this the gateway to inflammatory health: **live a good life, be happy, eat exceptionally and take care of your body.** Take in plenty of healthful and antioxidant foods or herbs. Immune strength and inflammation are connected: and emotions play a huge role in immunity. Therefore, in order to ward off inflammation in the best way possible, strive to be happy and healthy! It's secretly that simple—and yet, it's no secret at all.

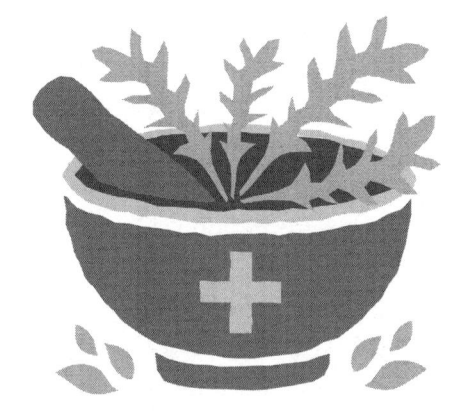

THANK YOU

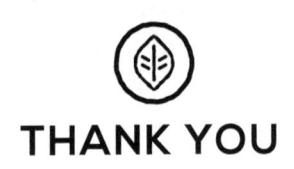

I'd like to thank you, again, for purchasing this book and exploring the amazing topics of health surrounding inflammation with me. I hope that my knowledge, research, and journey have given you some invaluable ideas and tips you can use to inform your own unique path—a path towards prime immune health, good diet habits, and the energy and wellness you so deserve, which can be so easily taken away by the subtle influence of chronic inflammation!

The world if information out there on inflammation can be confusing and overwhelming, but if you do feel lost in a sea of differing opinions, facts, and approaches—you can always turn to this book for comfort and knowledge again. Review the many foods to focus on, to get you back on track. Take a moment to look at the foods you should be steering clear of, or even give yourself a primer on the miracles of herbal medicine and supplements that can get you back to managing your inflammation in an exceptional, empowering way.

Remember: always use herbs and supplements in a cautious, informed way. Knowledge and self-education is power, and if you are ever in doubt about the state of your health and if inflammation is playing a role—never hesitate to contact a professional health practitioner who can help you with these issues, and helping you narrow down a cause or diagnosis. Especially if you fear that you face a major inflammatory disease.

I will leave you here, but stay connected and in touch with the *Carma Books* community for more books on holistic, natural, and plant-based health. Reach out again soon for forthcoming, much-talked-about health subjects, just like *Natural Anti-Inflammatory Remedies,* along with plenty of experiences and sharing of tips and knowledge on how to empower healing in your own life—and to get the most mileage out of your health potential!

Until next time, I wish you a wonderful, beautiful journey of your own, in happiness and health.

A WORD FROM THE PUBLISHER

Hi, I'm Carmen, a holistic health geek with a passion for health, herbalism, natural remedies, as well as whole-food and plant-based lifestyles. After resolving various health issues I have struggled with for many years, I aim to inspire and help improve your health and longevity by sharing the tireless hours of research and valuable information I have discovered throughout my journey. Through the power of nutrition and lifestyle, with an evidence-based approach, I believe you can achieve your health and wellness goals.

If you enjoyed this book, I would love to hear how it has benefited you and invite you to leave a short review on Amazon - your valuable feedback is always appreciated!

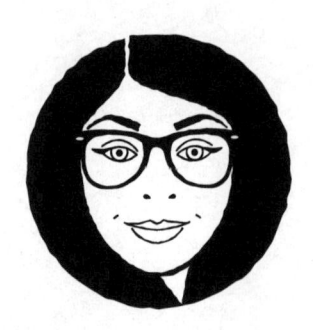

You are invited to to join our **Free Book Club** *mailing list. Sign up via our website to receive* **special offers** *and* **free for a limited time** *Health & Wellness eBooks!*

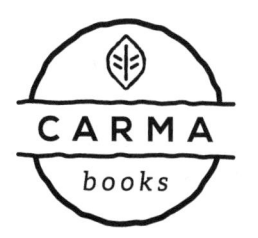

CARMA
books

'*A conscious approach to health & nutrition*'

carmabooks.com

THANK YOU

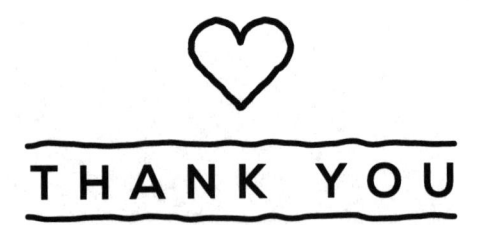

Made in the USA
Middletown, DE
03 February 2016